Harry HELPS Grandpa REMEMBER

BY KAREN TYRRELL

ILLUSTRATED BY AARON POCOCK

Published by Digital Future Press 2015

A catalogue record for this book is available from the National Library of Australia.

National Library of Australia Cataloguing-in-Publication entry:

Tyrrell, Karen, author
Harry Helps Grandpa Remember
Pocock, Aaron, illustrator

Book cover design and formatting services by BookCoverCafe.com

www.KarenTyrrell.com

First edition 2015

ISBN: 978-0-9872740-8-3 (pbk) 978-0-9872740-9-0 (e-bk)
978-0-9943021-2-0 (hbk)

The Regional Arts Development Fund is a Queensland Government through Arts Queensland and Logan City Council partnership to support local arts and culture.

Dedicated to Terrence Leo Tyrrell,

and Aubrey John Cox,

who inspired this story

Harry Hope lived happily on the
family farm with his mum and dad,
and his sister Sophie.

Grandpa and Nan lived in
their own house nearby.

Grandpa and Harry loved to play
hide-and-seek with Max the dog.

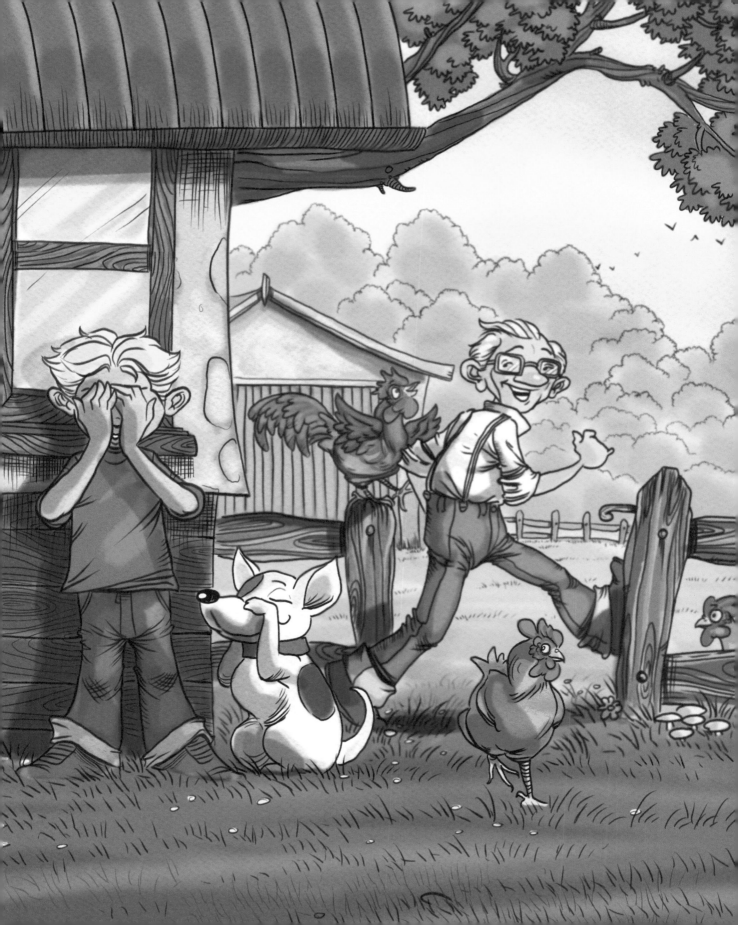

Harry began to notice that Grandpa
was getting slower, and he was
forgetting things.

One day Grandpa didn't want
to play with Harry anymore.

'I just want to rock in my rocking
chair,' grumbled Grandpa.

So Harry trudged home with Max.

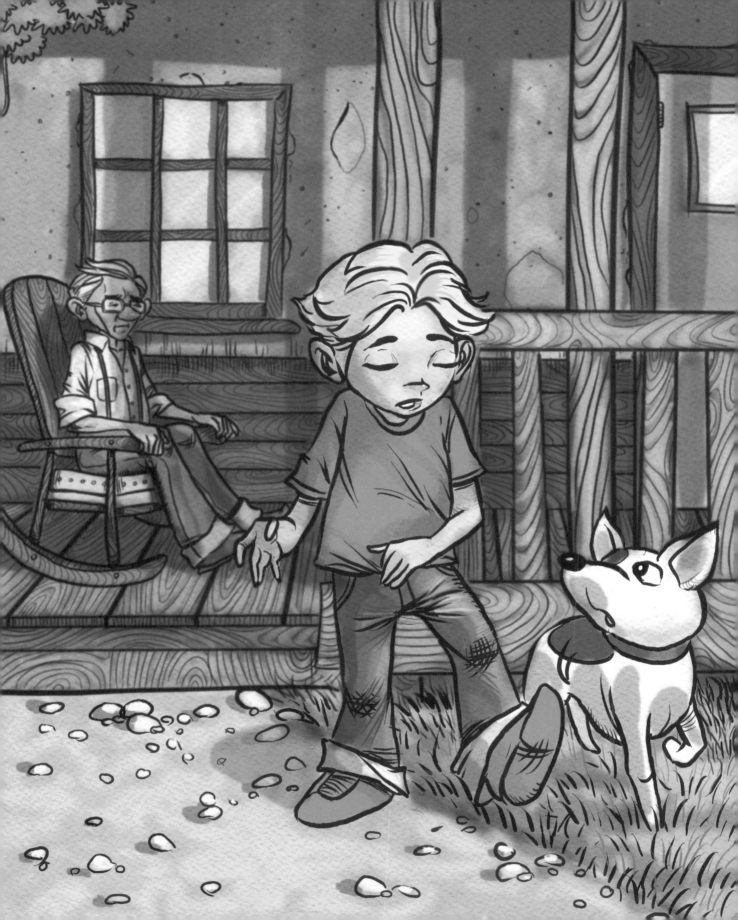

On Grandparents' Day at school,
Grandpa became confused and lost.

Harry and Nan found him sitting
all alone on a bench.

Harry was sad because Grandpa
had forgotten his name.

Nan hugged Harry. 'Grandpa is
getting very forgetful,' she said. 'We
must try to help him remember.'

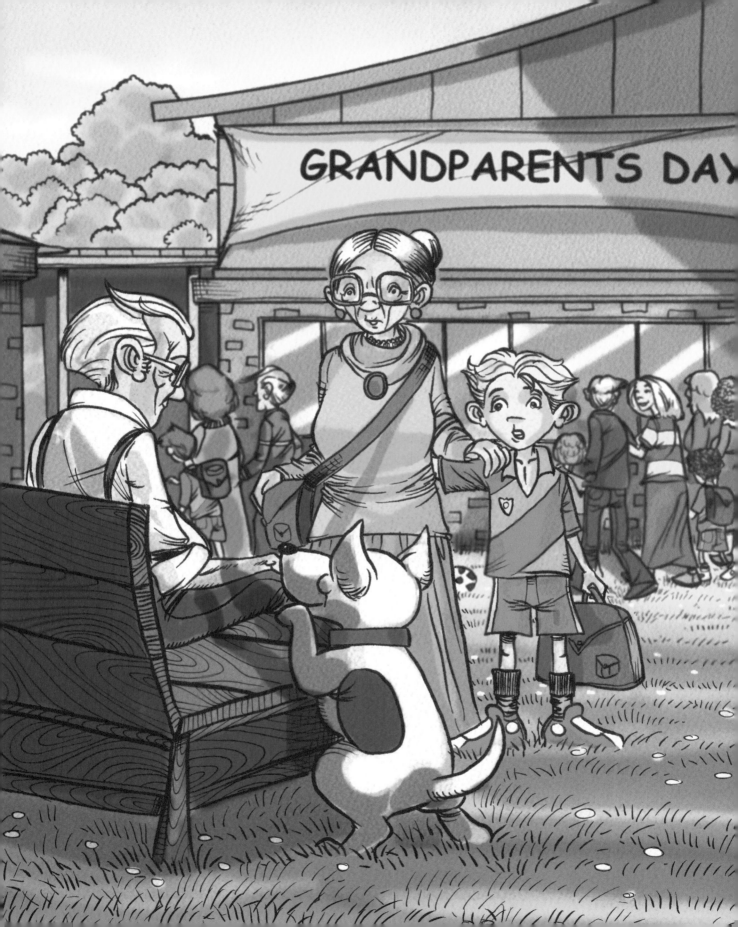

Harry thought of a wonderful idea
to help Grandpa remember.

He made Grandpa a diary with
reminders of all the things he had to
do on the farm.

Feed the chickens

Brush Neddy

Milk Daisy

Collect the eggs

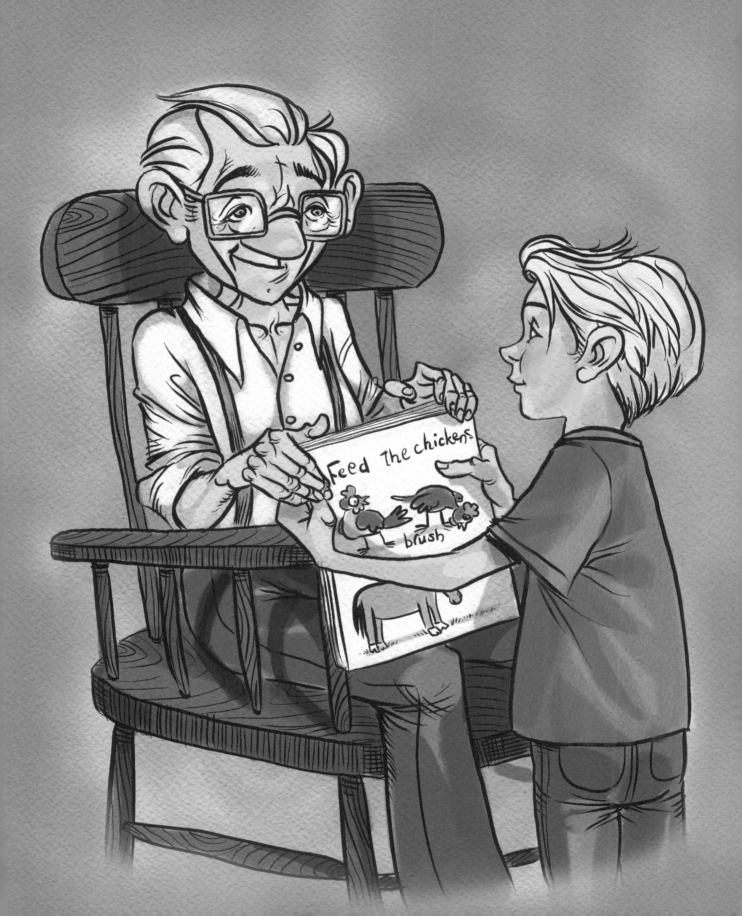

On Saturday, the family went to their favourite swimming hole.

Splish! Splash!

Dad hugged Harry and said, 'We'll treasure these memories forever.'

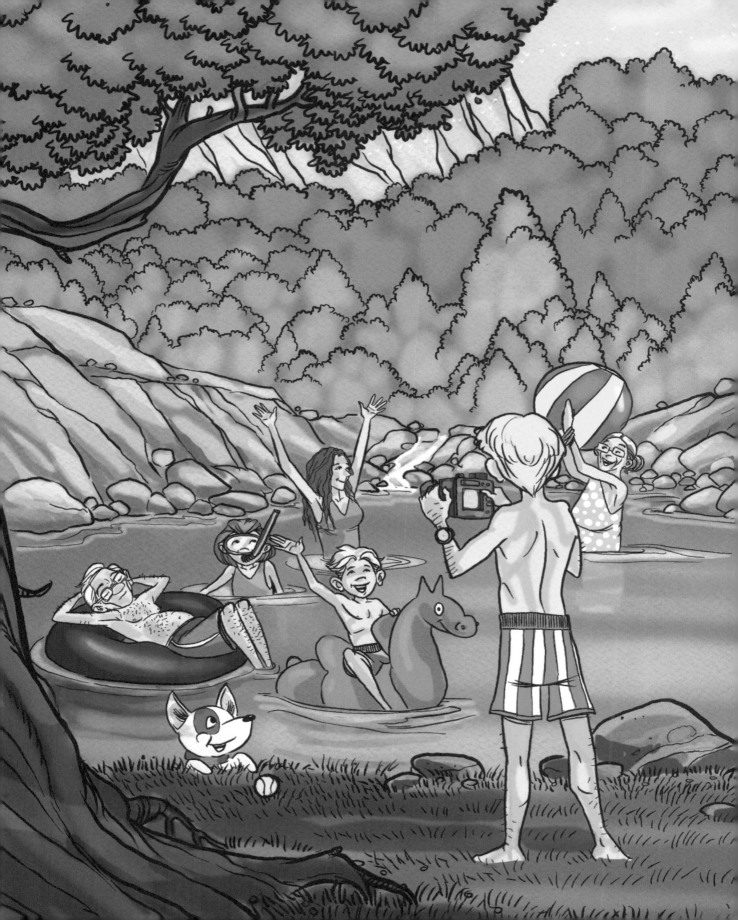

Harry thought of a wonderful way to make Grandpa's eyes twinkle.

'Do you have a photo album I could show Grandpa?' Harry asked Nan.

When Grandpa looked at a photo of him and Nan on their wedding day, Harry saw a sparkle in his eyes.

Grandpa flipped the pages, pointing and chuckling with Harry.

Grandpa

Nan

Grandpa and Nan on
their wedding day

Harry thought of a wonderful way
to make Grandpa smile.

He knew how much Grandpa loved all the
animals on the farm, so he said ...

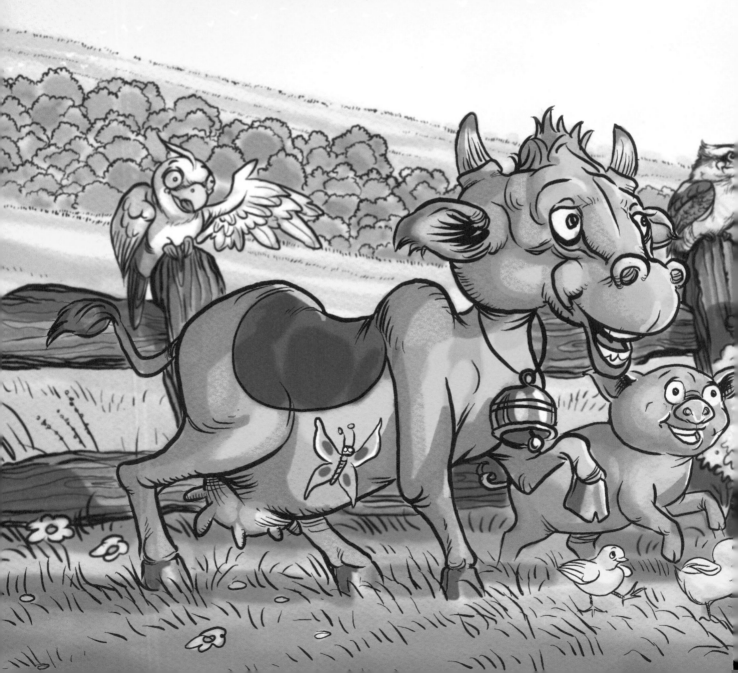

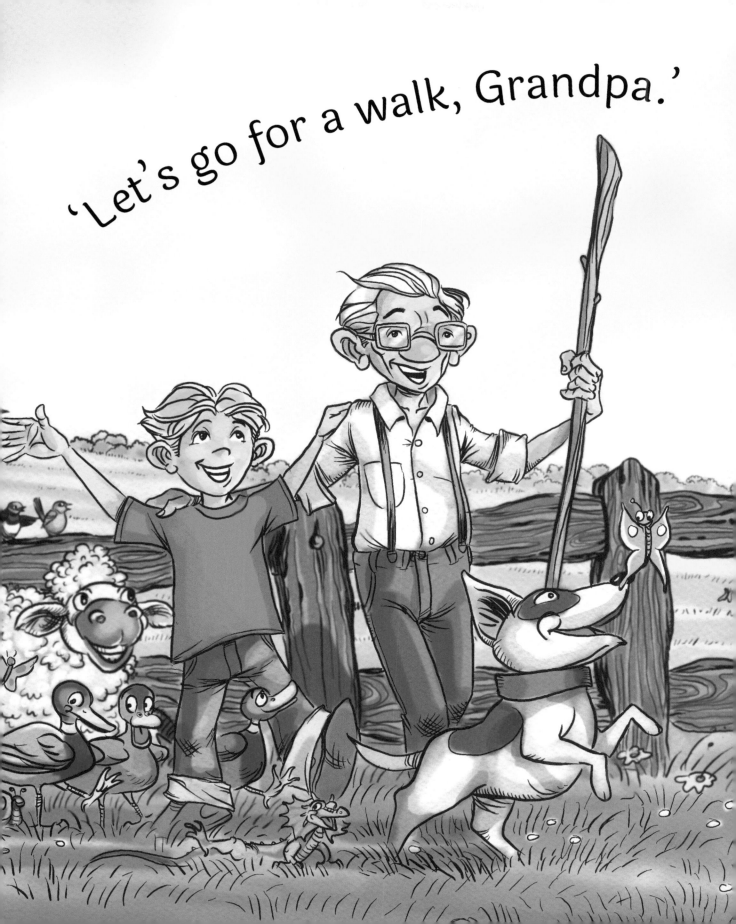

'Let's go for a walk, Grandpa.'

Miss Darling played her favourite
song from when she was a little girl.

'Oh,' she said with a sigh, 'how this
music makes me remember.'

Harry thought of a wonderful way
to make Grandpa laugh.

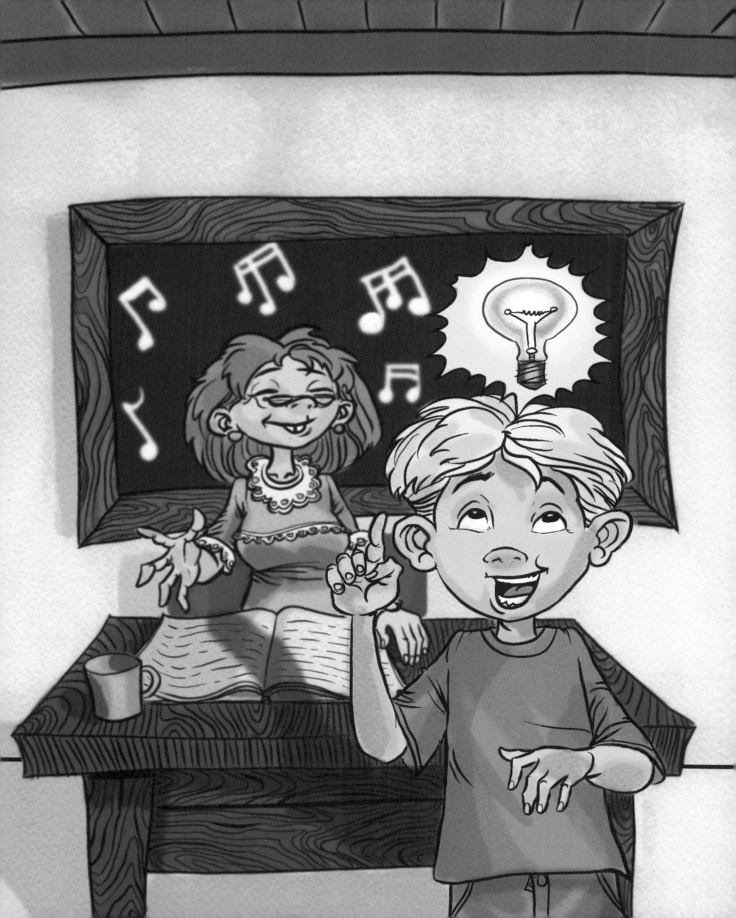

After school, Harry ran over to
Grandpa and Nan's house.

'Can you play Grandpa's favourite music?'
Harry whispered to Nan.

When he heard the music, Grandpa
laughed and tapped along
to the beat.

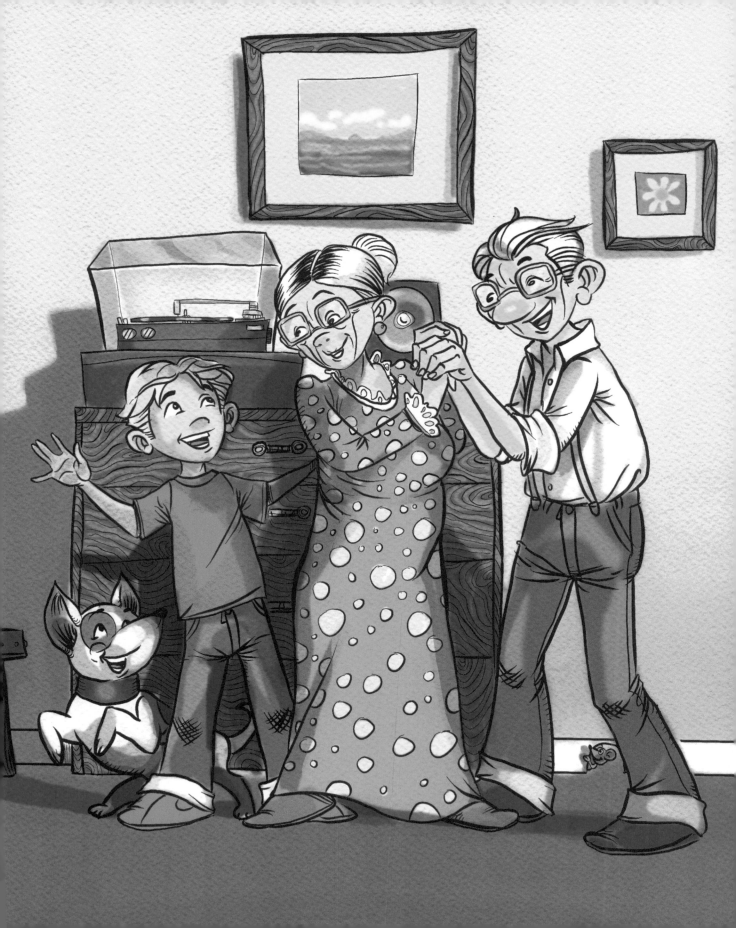

'What did Grandpa like to do
when he was young?'
Harry asked Nan.

'Why, Grandpa always loved
to bake,' said Nan.

Harry thought of a wonderful,
secret way to help
Grandpa remember.

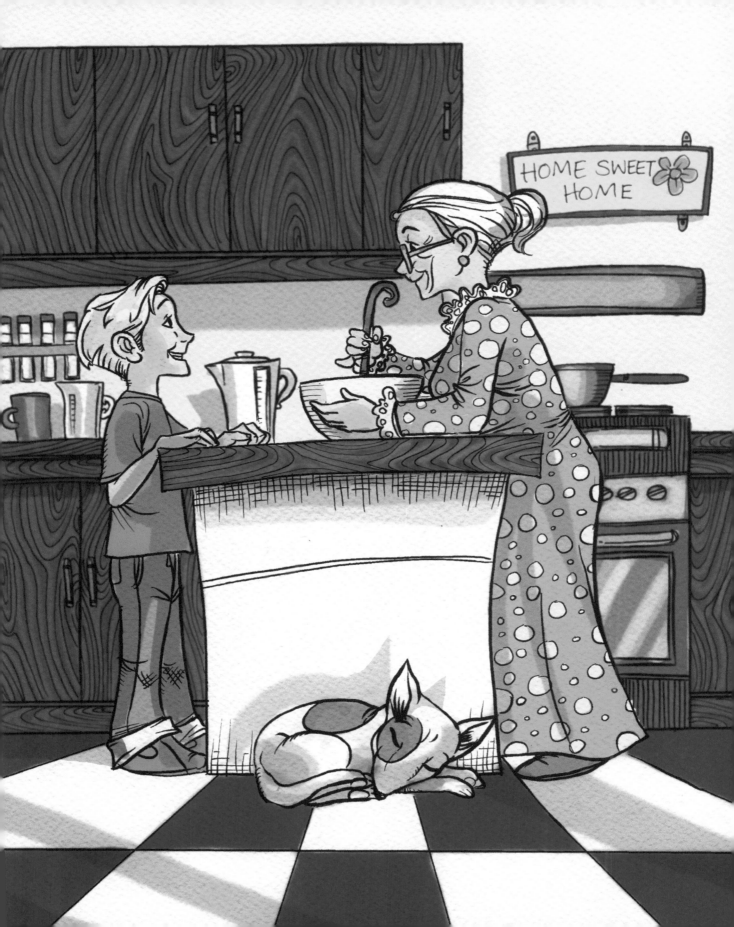

On Harry's birthday,
all Harry's friends arrived
to help him celebrate.

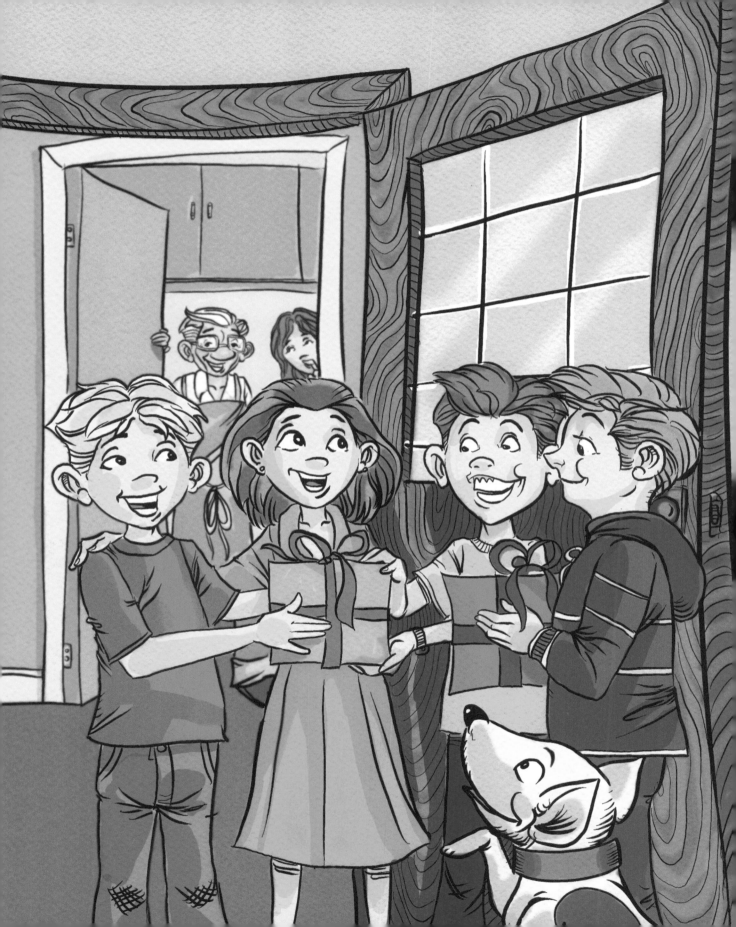

They played follow-the-leader,
and musical chairs,
and **lots** of other games.

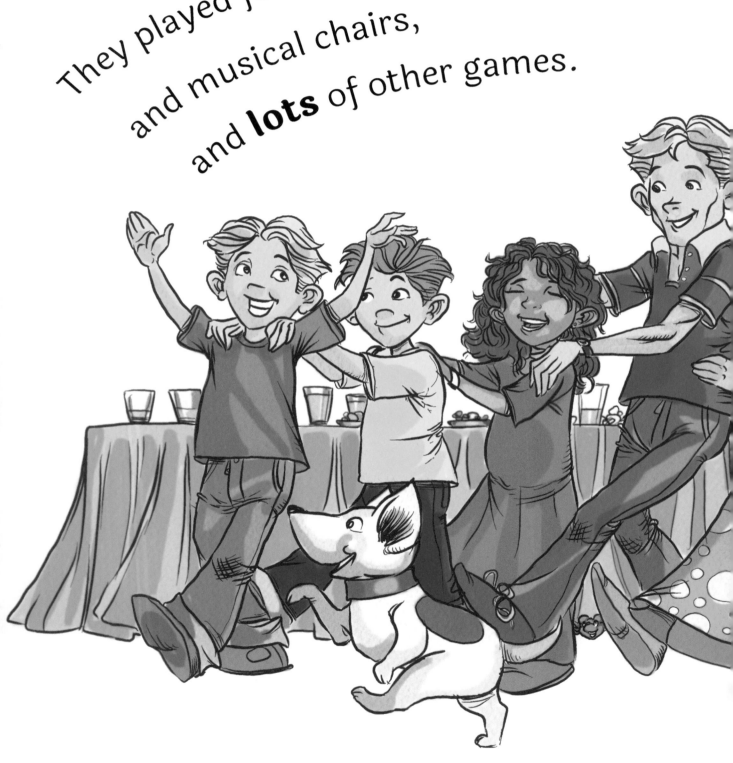

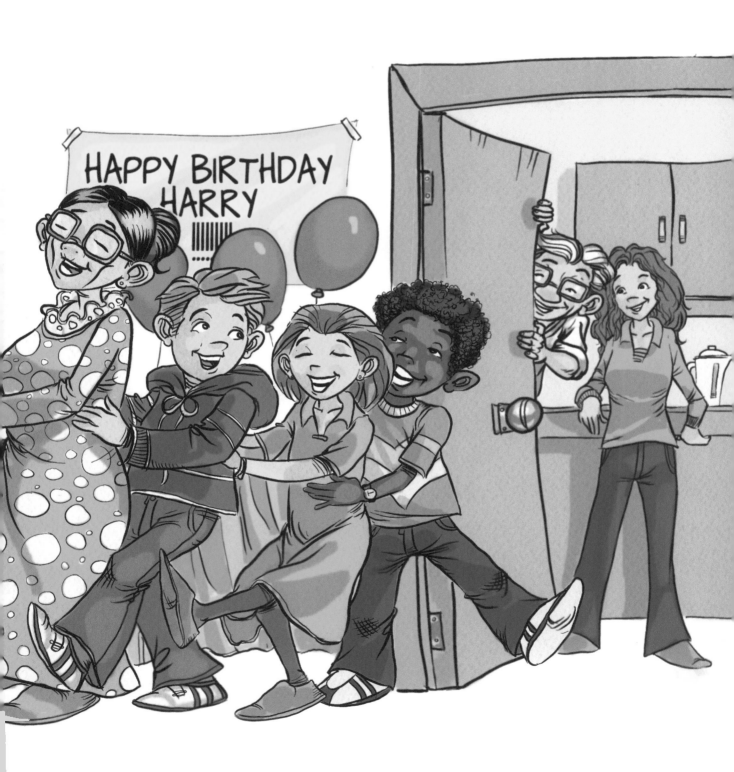

'Surprise!

Happy Birthday, Harry!'

said Grandpa.

Everyone sang 'Happy Birthday'.

Then they all gobbled up the
delicious chocolate cake
Grandpa had helped to bake.

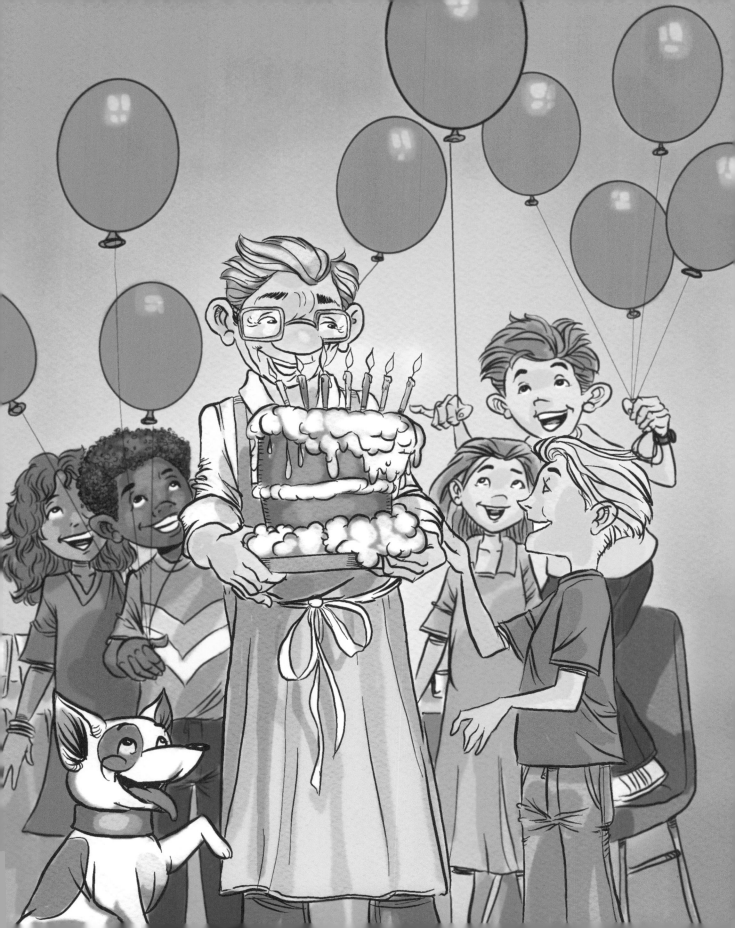

'What a wonderful party, Harry Hope,'
said Grandpa.

'You remembered my name, Grandpa.
This is the best birthday **ever**.'

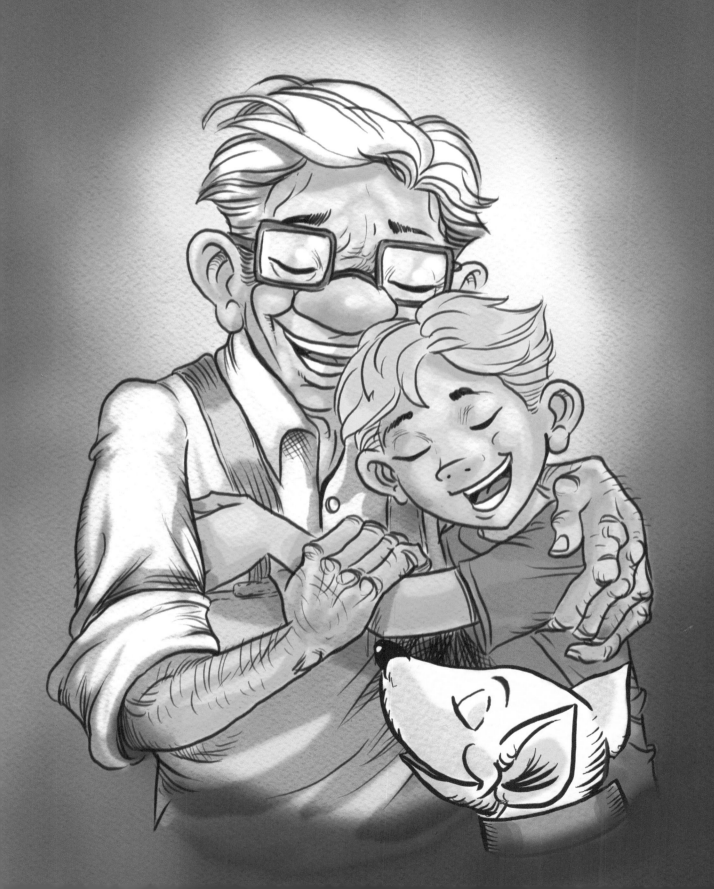

Note for Teachers & Families

Dementia, including Alzheimer's disease, affects people's memories and their powers of reasoning. Current research suggests that the risk of dementia may be reduced by taking the following steps:

1. Look after your heart.
2. Do some kind of physical activity each day.
3. Eat a healthy diet of fresh fruit and vegetables, and take fish oil.
4. Mentally challenge your brain with activities like crosswords and jigsaws.
5. Enjoy social activities.

For those already diagnosed with dementia, symptoms may be improved by calming daily routines, a healthy fresh diet, pet therapy, diary and whiteboard reminders, vivid nostalgic photos, music, dancing, singing, and physical activity.

Please contact your doctor for more information.

About the Author

Karen Tyrrell is an award-winning resilience author and teacher from Brisbane, Australia, who shares coping skills with children and families. Karen presents creative writing workshops and fun storytelling sessions at schools, libraries and festivals.

To discover more of Karen's books, free activities, and teacher resources visit KarenTyrrell.com.

Also by Karen Tyrrell:

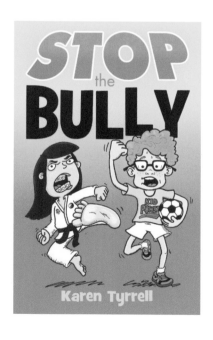

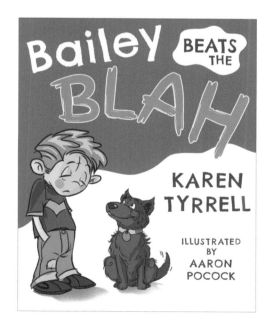